nine 2 five
yoga

Simple workplace exercises to ease and relieve the stress and tensions of your working day

Caroline Smart

D1196014

First published in 2004 by
New Holland Publishers (UK) Ltd
London * Cape Town * Sydney * Auckland

Garfield House, 86–88 Edgware Road
London W2 2EA
United Kingdom
www.newhollandpublishers.com

80 McKenzie Street
Cape Town 8001
South Africa

Level 1, Unit 4, 14 Aquatic Drive
Frenchs Forest, NSW 2086
Australia

218 Lake Road
Northcote, Auckland
New Zealand

ISBN 1 84330 698 0

Designed and created for New Holland Publishers by The Printer's Devil
Senior Editor: Clare Sayer
Production: Hazel Kirkman
Design: The Printer's Devil
Photographs: BlackEye Photography
except: Photodisk © pages 6 and 84

1 3 5 7 9 10 8 6 4 2

Reproduction by Modern Age Repro, Hong Kong
Printed and bound by Times Offset (M) Sdn. Bhd., Malaysia

WARNING

*When beginning any exercise routine, however gentle,
it is important to ensure that you are in good health.
Consult your doctor before you begin any exercise
programme, especially if you have a medical condition
or are pregnant. The author and publisher disclaim any
liability or loss, personal or otherwise, resulting from
any use of the procedures and information in this book.*

nine2five yoga: contents

nine2five yoga: introduction

You may be wondering how yoga and work can possibly mix. You may even have picked up this book out of curiosity, expecting to see advice on handstands at your desk or shoulder-stands in the boardroom. How could anyone do yoga in office clothes? And what will my colleagues say when they sees me sticking out my tongue and doing The Lion?

You needn't worry – the type of yoga we suggest is so subtle that many people will not even notice that you are doing it. But they might notice you are looking brighter, your posture is good and you are more focused at work. Just a few simple stretches, bends, twists and breathing exercises will give you a clearer sense of how you should sit, stand and move.

The exercises bring long-lasting benefits yet take only minutes. Following the routines in the book, you can practice:

- hand and wrist exercises daily, especially if you work at a keyboard;
- shoulder and neck exercises at least once a day, particularly if you have a sedentary job;
- eye exercises once or twice weekly if you work at a screen;
- leg exercises every day if your job doesn't let you get up and walk around as often as you would like;
- a twist a day – build it into your daily routine;
- complete breathing daily to focus your mind – you will feel the benefits especially if you work in a stressful environment.

Keep this book handy, on your desk or in a drawer, particularly for those times when you lapse! We all do. But once you have had a taste of the benefits of yoga, you will always come back. Remember, yoga is for everyone, anywhere, any time! This book will show you how to manage the part from 9 to 5.

what is yoga?

In General

What most people consider to be "yoga" is a gentle, if rather strange, form of physical exercise mainly done by women. These exercises often don't seem to involve very much movement or exertion and have odd-sounding names like "tree", "mountain" and "cowface". More confusing still, they also have a set of stranger, unpronounceable-looking names like *vrksasana*, *tadasana* and *gomukhasana*.

You may not realize that they are the same exercises, nor that yoga originated in India and that these strange names are the original Indian names, while "tree", "mountain", etc, are just translations into English from the Indian language, Sanskrit.

These exercises or poses (or *asanas*, in Sanskrit) are just one element of yoga. Other parts include breathing, meditation and diet. The ultimate aim of yoga is self-awareness or an understanding of your part in the great scheme of things. To embark on this journey towards understanding, bodies and minds must be healthy. You should also be able to concentrate and focus your mind.

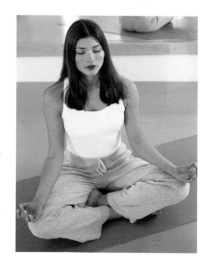

To reach this pure awareness, you have to filter out distractions. These come in many forms, and can be anything you like too much. For some it might be food, for others sex, others possessions and for most, laziness.

In this Book

Yoga can help free you from all of these distractions and correct any imbalances – that is, if you want it to. But you don't have to go the whole road. If you just want a strong supple spine, a flexible body and relaxed mind, you can stop there. The good thing is that once you have learned some of what yoga teaches you – for instance, how sitting badly affects you, or what effect tensing muscles that don't need tensing does to you – you cannot unlearn them. You can only go forward. So even if you do indulge in some bad habits, you can recognize them and know how to put them right. These good yoga habits stay with you and quietly nag you until you do sit up straight, you do pull your tummy in and you do lengthen the back of your neck.

Yoga is about balance, finding a balanced healthy way of life. If you have been to a class you will know that the exercises are also balanced: if you bend to the right, you repeat to the left; forward bends are followed by back bends; and energetic poses are counterbalanced by calming, quietening ones.

It is useful to bring this balanced approach to life into the office. An example of unbalanced activity is spending hours at a keyboard repeating the same movements with your fingers. If you don't counteract this with relief and rest to the hands, you might cause your body harm. This has been the case with the increasing incidences of Repetitive Strain Injury (RSI). You can prevent it, but once it happens it is very difficult to cure. Yoga can show you the way to take care of your body by taking this balanced approach to activity.

There are many forms of yoga and for those who want to explore all the different paths that yoga can take you on, there is an enormous amount of literature. We have included a list of further reading and interesting websites on page 93.

Why Bring Yoga into Work?

The simple answer to this is so that you can get more out of your work and be able to carry it out more efficiently so that it doesn't spill into your out-of-office life. Nowadays, office work often involves many hours sitting in front of a computer screen, perhaps in conditions which are not ideal: cramped space, badly ventilated rooms, bright harsh lighting, etc. Although yoga won't make your desk bigger or your computer faster or bring fresh air into your space, it can improve how you deal with the conditions around you, how you cope with your workload and how you deal with the stress of modern living.

Life is becoming more and more sedentary. We sit down for practically everything: from driving to work, to work itself, and for most forms of relaxation, and even going to the loo (no more squatting behind bushes!). We use our leg power less and less. And it is addictive. How many of us, when approaching a large shop which has a choice of automatic doors and ordinary swing doors, veer towards the automatic option? Even the simple of action of pushing or pulling becomes a chore when there is an electronic gadget that can do it for you.

In becoming more sedentary we lose strength in muscles that support the structure of our body. Tummies sag, spines slump and shoulders hunch. Sometimes we are unaware that this is happening, until we are thrown into a situation where, for example, we find ourselves sitting on the floor and our back is aching from sitting without the support of a chair back.

A few simple stretches and poses adapted to be done in an office environment can counter the effects of office life, and help improve your body (and mind!) at the same time.

counteracting the slump

REASONS WHY YOU SLUMP

- *you sit for too long at a desk.*
- *you wear high heels which throw your weight forward.*
- *you have a big bust and you let it drag you forward.*
- *over the years your belly has got bigger.*
- *you carry a heavy handbag and it pulls you to one side.*
- *you drive with your chin pointing upwards and you scrunch the back of your neck.*
- *you poke your head forward so your neck has to work to counteract the weight of your head.*
- *you have lost mobility in your shoulders, so you hunch forward.*
- *you have become muscle-bound and inflexible.*

Good posture is something that comes naturally when you learn to walk. Just watch toddlers sitting on the floor in front of the television. They sit perfectly straight, transfixed by what they are watching. Then look at a teenager sitting in the same position. It's unlikely that they are sitting beautifully straight, their backs are more likely to resemble a very curved banana, if they can bear to sit without support at all.

Toddlers seem to know instinctively how to hold their bodies. They bend their knees to pick up a toy and use the strength of their legs to support their own weight and the weight of what they are carrying. Unfortunately, years spent slumping forward at a school desk, and other accumulated bad habits, destroy the good posture we were born with.

However, the good news is that once you become aware of how best to stand and sit, you can relearn all the good stuff.

The Spine

The key to good posture is understanding the spine and how it is designed to work. It helps support the standing weight of your body and is the column on which your head sits. It bends backwards and forwards and can even twist in both directions at once. It protects and encloses the spinal cord which takes all the information from the brain to the various parts of the body telling them what to do. According to yoga, the spine is also the channel along which energy travels, and any blockages along its length can cause problems. For a fuller explanation of this, see page 84.

In yoga there is a saying, "you are as old as your spine", and the key to a long and healthy life is keeping your spine as flexible as possible. And although there may be some things you cannot avoid – such as arthritis or rheumatism – you can keep them at bay with regular movement and gentle exercise.

Let's look at the spine and see why it is such a remarkable feat of engineering and why we should take more care of it.

Because the spine has to move in all directions, it can't be made up of one rigid bone like the mast of a ship. To allow bending and twisting movements the spine is made up of over 30 small bones known as vertebrae, and so that they don't

COMMON CAUSES OF SPINE DISTORTION

- **Weak tummy muscles** mean that the spine is not supported properly and the lower spine is having to take on extra weight.

- **A large tummy** perhaps due to pregnancy or overindulgence in beer, pulls the small of the back forward, particularly when standing, and puts extra strain on this area.

- **Sway back** is where the pelvis and top of the hips are pushed forward and the upper body swayed back to counteract it. It can result in shortened muscles in the lower back. Any slight twist or sudden jerk of the lower back can cause acute pain in tight muscles.

- **Rounded shoulders** are where the ribcage is squashed, lungs constricted, and the back appears slightly humped. This is often made worse by long periods spent crouched at a desk.

grind together, they have pads between them made of cartilage and filled with a jelly-like substance. These pads or discs act as shock absorbers, protecting the spine from jarring when you walk or run or jump.

You might think that a straight spine should be ramrod-straight. However, you would be wrong. The spine has natural curves which provide additional give for movements like running and jumping. This give stops your spine from jarring.

The Correct Way To Stand

Good posture is a basic building block for good health. You'd think knowing how to stand would be easy, but it is surprising how many people are not sure how to stand correctly.

How do you stand?

These are some of the most common posture faults. Can you identify yourself in one of these postures?

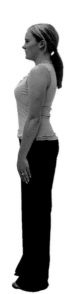

Sticky-out Bottom: Affects women who wear high heels and tip their weight forward. The pelvis tilts down and knees are pushed back (you may see it in young gymnasts). Too much curve at the small of the back results in tight back muscles and weak tummy ones.

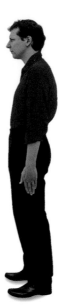

Military Man: The military look where the spine and rest of body is held too rigidly. Muscles are so tight that any jerk or twist can cause problems.

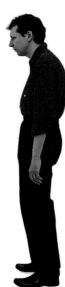

Concave Man: The droopy man look. He generally thrusts his pelvis forward so it tips up at the front (with hands in pockets) then hunches his spine forward, constricting his chest and abdomen. Tummy and shoulder muscles are weak. This is also known as Flat Back.

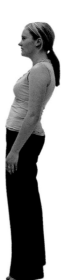

Swayback: Often affects pregnant women or men with beer bellies. The tummy is pulled forward and it pulls the lower spine with it. To compensate the top of the body is swayed back.

Correct your posture

Here is your good-posture checklist. Start from the feet and work your way up. As you check, feel as though you are growing tall through the soles of your feet.

- Have your feet about hip-width apart. Your feet should be pointing forward and parallel, i.e. the same distance runs between the inside edges of your feet.

- The weight of your body should be spread evenly across the soles of your feet.

- Feel as though you are lifting through the arches of your feet, not sinking under the weight of your body.

- Knees should be soft, don't lock them back.

- Feel your thigh muscles pulling up slightly

- The small of your back should feel as though it is being pressed against the wall behind you, reducing some of the curve in the small of your back. Your tailbone automatically tucks in.

- Tummy muscles should be pulled in to support your lower

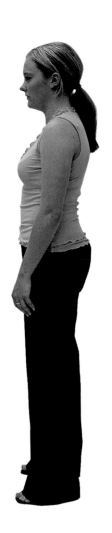

spine, you immediately feel trimmer and you can feel your spine lifting, growing taller.

- Shoulders should feel relaxed and down, with shoulder blades sliding closer together allowing your chest to open. Palms turned to the front will help open the chest.

- You should feel the back of your neck pressed towards the wall behind you so that it lengthens. Your chin should drop a fraction.

- Feel the crown of your head as the tallest point of your body. Imagine a golden thread pulling the crown of your head towards the ceiling.

Now check that with the effort involved in such a simple pose, you aren't tensing up parts of the body that don't need to be. Your jaw may have locked. Your eyes might be staring. Your tongue might be sticking to the roof of your tongue. Soften and relax any tension in your body.

The part the pelvis plays in good posture

"Pelvis" means "basin", and you should think of it as a basin that protects and supports the lower organs, including the bladder and the reproductive organs, as well as the developing baby in pregnant women.

The position of the pelvis is very important in good posture. Try to visualize it as a basin full of water. If the pelvis is tipped forward (water running out of the front), then it pulls the lower back too far forward and you compensate by throwing your upper body back (sway back). If it is tilted backward (water running out of the back), then it causes your lower back to slump. For perfect posture it should be tilted neither forward nor back (the water stays inside the basin). So whatever position you might be in (sitting, standing, on a bicycle), visualize that basin of water and keep your pelvis in its perfect (neutral) position.

The Correct Way To Sit

Now that you realize the importance of the natural curves of the spine and the neutral position of the pelvis, it will help you to sit properly.

Many problems associated with sitting at a desk for long periods come from poor posture. When you know how your body should be, you can check that the chair you are sitting on, the desk you are using and the screen you are staring at are all adjusted to ensure you are sitting correctly. Although RSI mainly affects your arms, wrists and fingers, the causes probably start with how you are sitting.

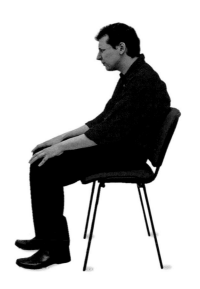

The illustrations show typical examples of poor seated posture: above, a slump; and below, overstretched on a chair that is too high.

Finding your sitting bones

You need to be sitting on your sitting bones. If you don't know where they are or you are well endowed in the rear you can find them by sitting on the floor and placing the palms of your hands beneath your buttocks (you may have to spread your buttocks a little). Then rock back and forth and feel for the bony bits that stick down. Slide your hands out and keep feeling the bony bits in contact with the ground.

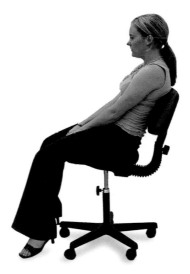

Now you are ready to sit tall.

- Feel the weight of your body spread evenly across your sitting bones.

- Feel your spine lengthening as you press the small of your back towards the wall behind you.

- You should feel your tummy muscles kicking in to support your spine.

- Shoulders should be down and relaxed. Shoulder blades slide down and towards each other, opening your chest to the front.

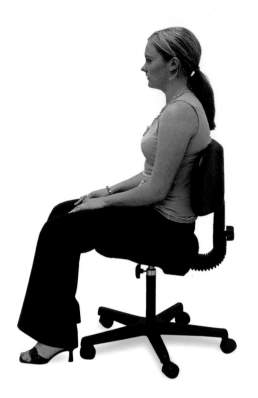

The correct way to sit

- Feel as though you are pressing the back of your neck against the wall behind you and look straight ahead.

- Your chin drops naturally and imagine the crown of your head being pulled toward the ceiling by a golden thread.

Pelvic rocking

You need to be sure that your pelvis is in the correct position. No spilling the water in your pelvic basin! To get a feel of how the position of your pelvis can affect how you sit, try some pelvic rocking.

From your sitting position on the floor, rock backwards off your sitting bones. Did you feel the small of your back slump? Rock forwards off your sitting bones. Did you feel the small of your back curve too far forward, causing the top part of your body to sway backwards? That's bad pelvic rocking.

Now try some good rocking. This is how to do it right.

Sit correctly as described above. Then move your pelvis backward and forward just to ease out the small of your back. Visualize that basin of water and swish the water back and forth. But don't let it spill out!

Once you have become familiar with your pelvis, you can practise the pelvic rocking sitting, standing or lying down.

It's a great way of easing any lower-back pain.

Forward Arm Stretch

Interlock your fingers and straighten your arms out in front of you with palms facing out.

You should feel the stretch in the arms and shoulder blades.

Hold for two breaths and repeat.

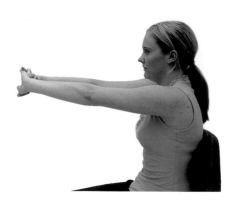

Vertical Arm Stretch

Interlock your fingers and, turning palms, stretch your arms above your head so that they are straight.

Hold for a breath, relax, and hold for another breath.

Repeat twice.

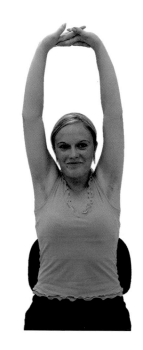

Sideways Stretch

1 Take your arms over your head and take hold of the outside of your left hand with your right hand.

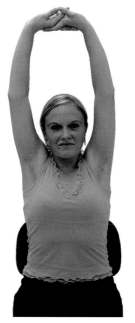

2 Pull your left arm to the right side. Keep arms as straight as you comfortably can and turn your chest slightly to the ceiling. You should feel a stretch along your left side. Hold for two breaths.

Repeat on other side.

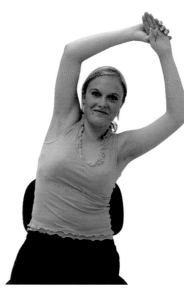

Upper-Arm Stretch

1 Hold your right elbow with your left hand (your right hand should hang down between your shoulder blades as in the illustration below) and pull your right elbow behind your head. You will feel the stretch in the back of the upper arm.

2 Hold for three breaths (but do not strain).

Repeat on other side.

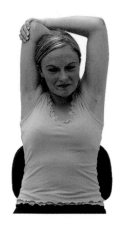

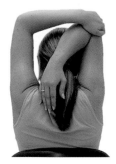

Upper-Arm Stretch & Twist

1 Hold your right arm above the elbow with your left hand.

2 Gently pull your elbow towards your left shoulder and turn your head slowly to look over your right shoulder.

Hold for two breaths. Repeat on other side.

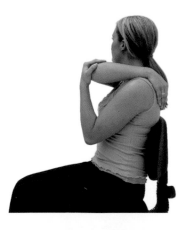

Forearm Stretch

1 Place palms of your hands flat on your chair on either side of your hips. Palms should be flat, fingers pointed backwards so that thumbs are to the outside.

2 Slowly lean arms back to stretch the forearms.

Hold for two breaths.

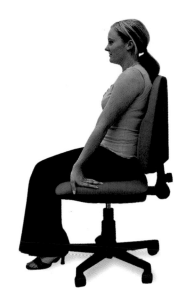

Lower-Back Stretch

This stretch is good because it is practically an upside-down pose where your head is lower than your heart, so fresh blood flows down to the brain. Avoid if you have high blood pressure.

1 Relax the front of your body down between your legs with arms hanging down.

2 Keep your bottom on the seat and release any tension in the small of your back.

3 Hold for five breaths. To come up, place your hands on your thighs and push body upright.

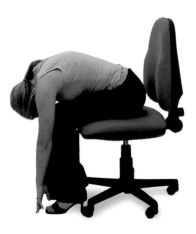

Chest Expander

If you sit hunched at a desk for several hours a day, this movement is ideal to help loosen tension in your shoulders. You can do this exercise standing or sitting.

1 Stand with your feet flat on floor slightly apart and parallel. If you are sitting, sit on the edge of your chair and press lightly down on the soles of your feet.

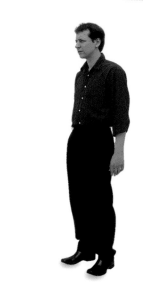

2 Straighten your spine: feel as though you are trying to press the small of your back against the wall behind you. Relax your shoulders and lengthen the back of your neck. (Imagine you are pressing the back of your neck against the wall behind you. Your chin will drop a fraction and the crown of your head will be the tallest point of your body).

3 Lift both arms straight out in front of you.

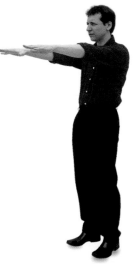

4 Swing them both round behind you at shoulder height, interlocking fingers (palms facing inward).

5 Breathing in deeply, squeeze your shoulder blades together. Try to straighten your elbows and imagine they are trying to touch one another. (If you are sitting, make sure the back of the chair isn't stopping you do this!)

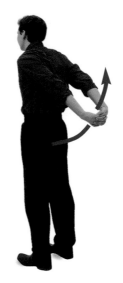

6 Breathing out, begin to lengthen forward, your head moving slowly forwards, stretching out your spine. Imagine your head is being pulled away from your hips.

7 When your upper body is parallel with the floor, bring your interlocked hands/arms as far forward over the top of your head as possible. You may find you cannot take them very far over at first but with practice you will soon loosen up this area.

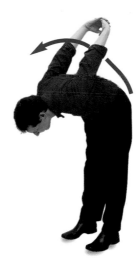

8 Breathing in, return to an upright position. Release your hands/arms and repeat the exercise at least three times. You should gradually feel more movement across the backs of the shoulders.

nine2five yoga

The Blade

Improves bustline and pectoral muscles. Relieves tension.

1 Sit or stand with arms extended out to the side at shoulder height; palms face downwards.

2 Pull your shoulder blades together as though you were trying to hold a coin between them (see the photograph below). Don't do this by moving your arms backwards, but let your muscles do the work. Your arms and shoulders will come back automatically.

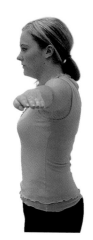

Repeat as many times as is needed to get rid of tension.

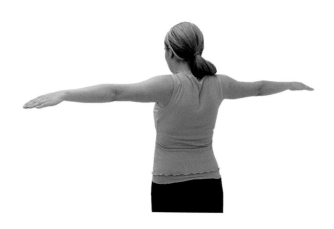

Shoulder Flexing

Relieves tension in the neck, back and shoulders. Increases lung capacity. Prevents dowager's hump.

1 Place fingertips on shoulders with elbows bent in front of you. Breathe in.

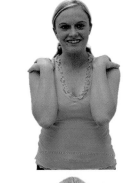

2 Breathing out, drop your chin to your chest and bring your elbows together in front of your body.

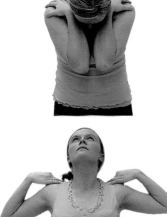

3 Breathing out, lift your head up and back, drawing your elbows back as though they want to touch behind your back.

Get into a rhythm and repeat ten times.

Cowface

Done sitting or standing, this is great for stiff shoulders and necks.

1 Sit on the edge of your chair, feet parallel, flat on floor and about a foot apart. Lift out of sitting bones. Feel as though you are trying to press the small of your back against the wall behind you; your shoulders are relaxed and down, the back of your neck long. (Imagine you are pressing the back of your neck against the wall behind you. Your chin will drop a fraction and the crown of your head will be the tallest point of your body).

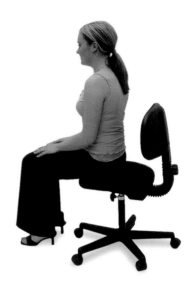

2 Take your left hand behind your back, palm outwards. Encourage it as high up between your shoulder blades as you can (use your other arm to help it up). Keep your left shoulder back and down.

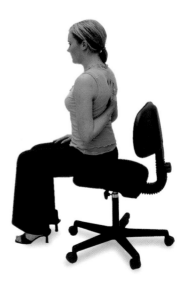

3 Breathe in and raise your right hand up to the ceiling. Then relax all of your right side on an out breath

4 Breathe in and begin to stretch through the right side of your waist, your armpit, elbow, wrist, fingers. Stretch towards the ceiling.

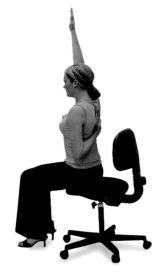

5 Breathe out and drop your right hand down behind you to clasp hold of the waiting left fingers. Keep shoulders and elbows back.

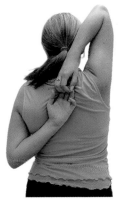

6 Hold for two breaths, unclasp hands and repeat on the opposite side.

TIP *If you find that you cannot reach, hold a tie or belt or scarf in the top hand and let it hang down so that the lower hand can catch hold of it. Try moving hands closer together using it and you should improve the looseness of your shoulders.*

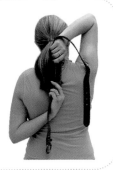

Chair Twist

Twists are movements that you might not do in everyday situations, yet they are wonderful for the spine, and it is well worth the effort incorporating them into your daily routine. Think of a twist as wringing out a wet sponge, getting rid of all the water. As soon as the spine straightens again, fresh blood rushes along its length, bathing all the nerve endings. Internal organs get a squeeze too!

Remember, you have to do it to both sides and you can even have a double twist, where you turn the neck and head the opposite way to the lower twist.

You have to do this on a chair with no arm rests.

1   Sit on the chair so that your legs are over the side and your right hip is as close into the chair back as possible; your bottom should be near the far edge of the seat. Make sure you are sitting tall, small of back pressed towards the wall behind you, shoulders relaxed and down, back of your neck long.

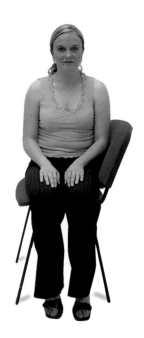

2 Breathing in, turn to face over the chair back, taking hold of each side. You should feel the spine twisting from the bottom up. See if you can have your shoulders in line with the back of the chair.

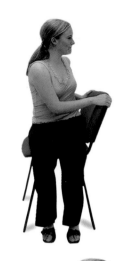

3 Stay like that and breathe out, turning your head directly over your shoulder in the direction in which you turned. You can push against the chair with your hands to get further into the twist.

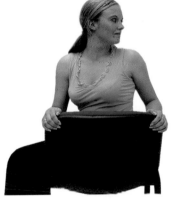

4 Breathing in, slowly turn your head to look the opposite way. Try not to lose height in the spine. It's just your head and neck that move.

Repeat on the opposite side, placing your left hip against the back of the chair.

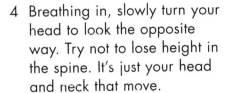
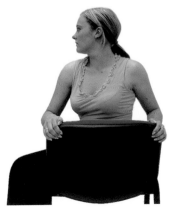
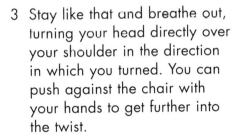

Bust Improver

If you do this correctly, you will feel the stretch on the upper bust.

1 Sit with your fingers interlocked behind your head.

2 Breathing in deeply, raise your hands up and back until your elbows are straight.

Hold for a couple of breaths.

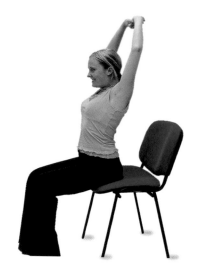

Chest Opener

1 Sit on the edge of your chair and take hold of the sides of the seat.

2 Breathing in, open your chest to the ceiling and drop your head gently back. (Imagine you have a loo roll wedged behind your neck.)

3 Stay like that for a couple of breaths feeling your chest open.

4 On an out-breath return to the starting position.

Repeat two or three times.

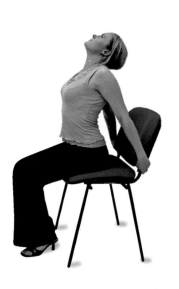

Sitting Forward Bend

1 Sit on the edge of the chair. Your legs should be straight out in front of you with your heels resting on the ground.

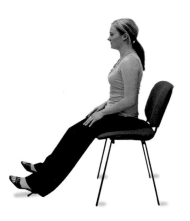

2 Breathe in and begin feeling some movement in your lower back as you take your chest towards the floor. Your arms move with you. Keep your head in line with your spine.

3 When you reach the end of the out breath, pause for a moment; you're in no hurry.

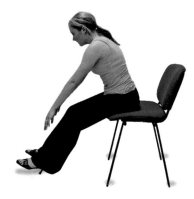

4 Breathe in and focus on your lower spine. Breathing out, continue moving forward.

5 When you have reached as far as you can, relax and breathe deeply.

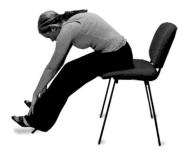

6 Breathing in, return upright. Feel as though the air in front of you is pushing your body back upright.

Repeat once or twice.

neck, shoulders & back

Keep those Shoulders Down!

If you aren't sure where your shoulders should be in terms of your posture, try this exercise.

All the exercises in this section can be done either standing or sitting.

How to Stand

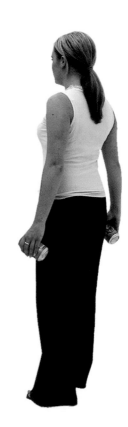

1 Take a drinks can in each hand and stand as described on pages 13–14.

2 Open your chest and feel your shoulder blades being pulled down and together by the weight of the cans. Get a feeling for this openness of the chest and put the cans down. Can you recreate the feeling and understand which muscles are working to keep your shoulders in that position? Whenever you find your arms dragging your chest forward, pick up the cans and recreate the feeling in your shoulders.

Up and Down

The nerves that connect the limbs and the body's different organs go through the neck. The neck and shoulders can become a hotspot for tension, especially if you spend a long time at a desk.

1 Begin with the back of your neck long and relaxed. Your chin will be tucked in slightly. Breathe in.

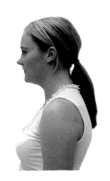

2 Breathing out, drop your chin onto your chest, feeling the stretch over the back of your neck.

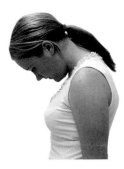

3 Breathing in, take your nose slowly up to the ceiling. Don't scrunch up the back of your neck. Imagine a loo roll is wedged there. Feel the stretch over the front of your neck.

Continue four times, dropping your head on an out-breath and lifting it on an in-breath.

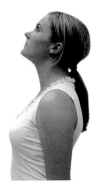

Side to Side

1 Begin with the back of your neck long and relaxed. Your chin will be tucked in slightly. Breathe in.

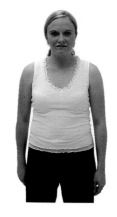

2 Breathing out, turn your head slowly to the right. Shoulders should stay down and relaxed. Only your neck and head move. Breathe in and return to the centre.

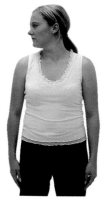

3 Breathing out, turn your head slowly to the left. Breathe in and return to the centre.

Continue four times each side, breathing out as you turn to each side and breathing in as you return to the centre.

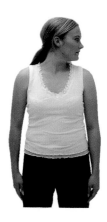

Ear to Shoulder

1 Begin with the back of your neck long and relaxed. Your chin will be tucked in slightly. Breathe in.

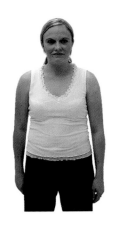

2 Breathing out, drop your right ear to your right shoulder. Feel the stretch across the left side of your neck. Don't be tempted to move your shoulder up to meet the ear. Breathe in and return to the centre.

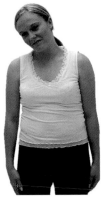

3 Breathing out, drop your left ear to your left shoulder. Feel the stretch across the right side of your neck. Breathe in and return to the centre.

Continue four times on each side.

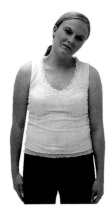

Head Circles

1 Begin with the back of your neck long and relaxed. Your chin will be tucked in slightly. Breathe in.

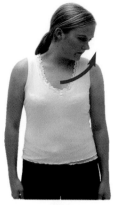

2 Breathe out and drop your chin to your chest.

3 Take your head round in three wide circles, then switch direction and go round the opposite way for three circles.

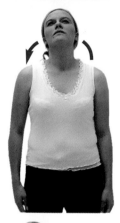

Don't drop your head too far back – imagine a loo roll is wedged at the back of your neck.

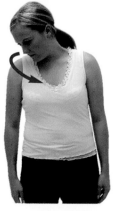

Shoulder Circles

1 Begin with the back of your neck long and relaxed. Your chin will be tucked in slightly. Breathe in.

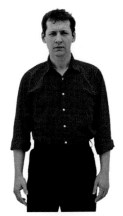

2 Make three large forward circles with your shoulders.

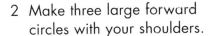

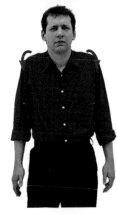

3 Switch direction and make three large backward circles with your shoulders.

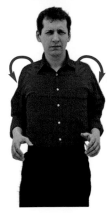

the energy of the hands

Yoga is about finding a healthy balance in your life. You may not be able to change the way you have to live your life: if your job involves sitting at a keyboard for hours on end, it is unlikely that you can change that. But you can change the way you approach your work, making sure you give your body a chance to cope with the lifestyle you are demanding of it. You and your body have to work together to make sure that you counterbalance the demands of your job, so that your work is done efficiently, but not at the cost of a fit, happy body.

Humans were not designed to sit rigidly in one position for many hours each day, making millions of tiny movements with fingertips on a keyboard. It is important to bear this in mind, particularly when you have a stressful job which means that you might be inclined to compromise your health for the sake of getting the work done.

RSI (Repetitive Strain Injury)

You may be someone, or know someone who suffers from carpal tunnel syndrome, or the more generally termed RSI, which includes things like tennis elbow. You don't have to be a keyboard operator to get it – it affects anyone whose work involves repetitive movement of the hands, doing the same task over and over again for several hours a day, from musicians through hairdressers to assembly-line workers. And once you have got it, you are more or less stuck with it. Although you can control it, it is extremely difficult to cure. The good news is that it is simple to prevent.

DON'T IGNORE THE RSI WARNING SIGNALS!

- *Any discomfort in your fingers, hands, wrists and arms, including tingling, numbness, weakness.*
- *Shooting pains in fingers, thumbs, wrists, elbows and arms.*
- *Tennis elbow or tendinitis.*
- *Difficulty performing everyday tasks, such as doing up buttons, twisting open lids, brushing teeth and opening or closing doors.*

What causes RSI?

The causes of RSI, or carpal tunnel syndrome, are not fully understood. It is believed that it is caused by pressure on the median nerve which goes from the forearm to the hand through a "tunnel" in the wrist, made up of the wrist bones and ligaments. Through this "tunnel" run tendons that connect to the finger and thumb bones. By continually constricting this area (perhaps from holding arms and hands in awkward positions), both muscles and tendons become strained and circulation is reduced. This can result in tiny tears which become inflamed. If this is ignored, and you do not rest the area, then scarring can occur restricting the blood circulation and causing further damage. Throw in a bit of stress and tension to wreak further havoc in your upper body, and the damage is done.

How to avoid RSI

The real key to avoiding these types of injury is understanding what an important part posture plays. You could have the most ergonomically equipped office in the world, but if you don't understand why you need it, you are unlikely to use it properly.

Likewise, you need to understand your body. It isn't designed to sit all day and stare fixedly at a screen. You have to give it breaks, let it stretch now and again, indulge in the odd twist and rest your eyes from over-stimulation.

The following are the points that you must remember. You could copy them onto a card and pin them up somewhere near your screen so that they don't just slip your mind when your boss is demanding those end-of-year figures.

How Flexible Are You?

This will give you an idea of how flexible your body is.

1 Place the palms of the hands together, as though you were saying a prayer.

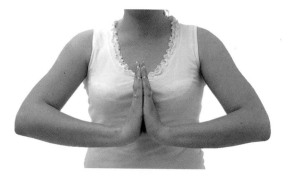

2 Press the fingers of both hands against each other. Your fingers should easily and painlessly bend back at right angles to the palm.

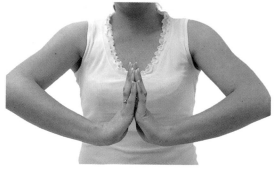

THINK PERFECT!

P Posture: make sure you are sitting correctly. Pelvis should be in neutral with spine lifting upwards. Shoulders should be down and sliding back. The back of your neck should be long with chin down slightly. The crown of your head is the tallest point. When you are tired, you slump, so get up, walk around and take a break.

E Exercise: do the wrist, hand and finger exercises before you begin work and during the day. Also do the eye exercises and practise Palming (see page 58) if you are spending particularly long stretches at the screen. And remember to stretch your upper body.

R Rest: take frequent rest breaks from the keyboard (5–10 minutes every hour), getting up and leaving your desk. Use breaks to do shoulder and neck exercises (see page 32).

F Feet: check that both your feet are flat on the ground. If not, adjust your chair or get a footstool.

E Elbows: tuck in your elbows close to your sides with forearms and hands at right angles to your body and resting on the desk. Remember to straighten out your elbow joints a few times during the day.

C Chair: make sure that your chair is adjusted to the proper height so that your thighs are horizontal and that the back-rest provides support to your lower back.

T Tension: often a cause of hunched shoulders and neck. Be aware of any tension in your upper body and practise the different stretches to keep muscles loose and relaxed (see pages 22, 24 and 26). Spend a few moments breathing properly (see page 78), and breathe away any tension.

Arm Energy Builder

This pose builds up the strength of the arms and hands, toning the muscles and nerves of the arms. It doesn't build muscle bulk, but increases the energy flow so that your arms grow strong and do not tire easily. However, you must practise it with awareness to stimulate the energy to flow correctly through your arms, wrists and hands.

1 Begin with your right palm facing forward and tucked into your right armpit.

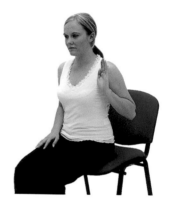

2 With the heel of your hand leading, push the air forward until your right arm is straight.

3 Return the hand to the starting position and repeat for a total of seven times.

Repeat the same movement with your left hand seven times. Breathe smoothly and slowly throughout.

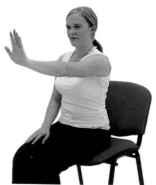

TIP *There should be no heaviness in these movements. Feel the warmth and energy in your hands as you push the air forward. Check that you don't build any tension in your hands and wrists.*

Hand & Wrist Exercises 1

- Elbows tucked into your sides, holding your hands out in front of you, wrists limp, shake your hands loosely ten times. Feel as though you are shaking water from your fingertips.

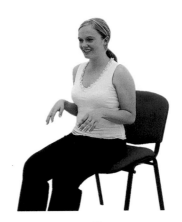

- Elbows tucked into your sides, holding your hands out in front of you, make loose fists and then stretch out your fingers, getting as much space between your fingers as possible. Don't over-tense the fingers.

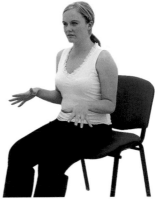

- Elbows tucked into your sides, holding your hands out in front of you, wrists limp, rotate both hands five times in one direction and then five times in the opposite direction.

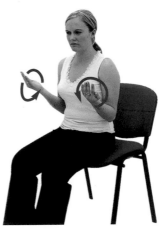

Hand & Wrist Exercises 2

- Elbows tucked into your sides, palms together in a prayer pose and keeping fingertips touching, push your hands open. Keep pressing fingertips firmly for 10 seconds. Relax hands together and repeat.

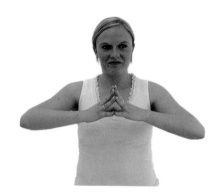

- Elbows tucked into your side, hold your hands out in front of you, palms down, and beginning with thumbs and index fingers touching, flick each finger away in turn. Then reverse back from the little fingers.

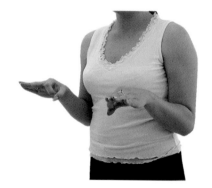

- Forearms resting on your desk, fingers soft and relaxed, keep your little fingers in contact with the desk, roll your hands outwards so that both palms face the ceiling. Roll the hands back inwards.

Repeat several times.

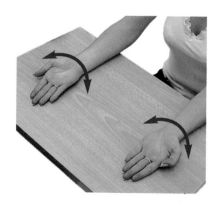

Ball Squeeze

You will need a soft rubber ball about 6 cm (2½ in) across.

1 Cup the ball in your right hand and squeeze it with all your fingers and thumb. Do it until your hand gets tired. Pause for a moment or two and repeat for a few more squeezes.

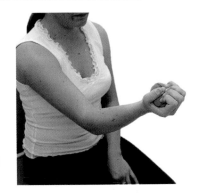

Repeat the squeeze with your left hand.

2 With your right hand, hold the ball between your little finger and thumb and squeeze ten times. Then do it with your ring finger and thumb, your middle finger and thumb and index finger and thumb. Squeeze ten times with each.

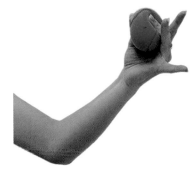

Repeat the squeezes with your left fingers and thumb.

3 Once you have completed the above squeezes, stretch open your hands one at a time. Separate and stretch your fingers. Concentrate on stretching, not tensing.

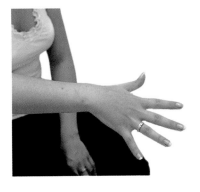

Up and Down Hands

1 Stretch your arms straight out in front of you. Palms face down and fingers point forward.

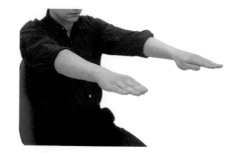

2 Bend hands back so that fingers point towards the ceiling. Palms push towards the wall in front of you.

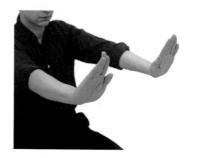

3 Bend hands down so that fingers point towards the floor, the backs of hands pushing towards the wall in front of you.

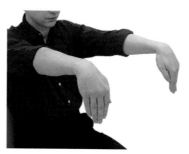

Repeat each movement seven times.

Keyboard Warm-ups

> Do these before you begin any long stretches at the keyboard.

- Open and close your fist a dozen times. Stretch out (but don't tense) fingers and thumbs as wide as possible.

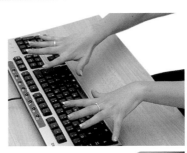

- Make loose fists and make slow circles with your wrist five times in one direction, then five times in the other.

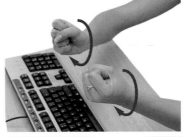

- With wrists bent and palms forward, press the top half of the fingers into the edge of the desk. Repeat several times.

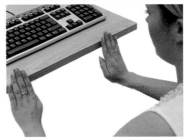

- With elbows bent, and hands at shoulder level, shake your hands as though you were shaking water from your fingers. Shake away any tension and tiredness in your hands.

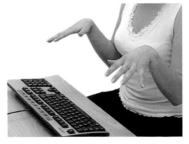

Finger & Hand Massage

1 Using the other hand, slowly rotate the thumb and all the fingers in turn on each hand. Do the rotation in both directions.

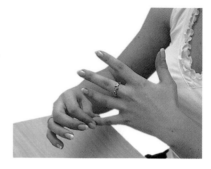

2 Bend each finger twice. First bend the top two joints by using the thumb of the opposite hand to press down the top of each finger joint.

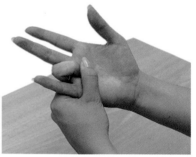

3 Then, keeping the finger straight, bend it down at the knuckle joint so that it lies flat on the palm.

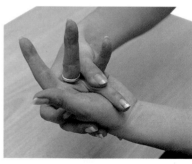

4 Making a fork with the index and middle finger of one hand, bend back each finger of the opposite hand in rapid succession. The angle of the bend should be 90° (less indicates stiffened joints).

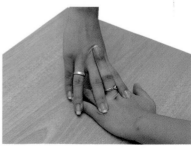

Finger & Thumb Stretch

1 Each finger at a time, gently stretch them backwards with the opposite hand. Then stretch all the fingers back at the same time.

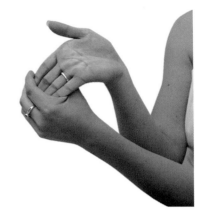

2 Bend your thumb gently back towards your wrist, but be careful not to overdo it. Then gently bend it forwards towards your wrist.

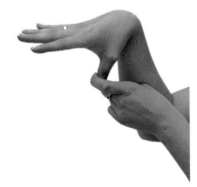

3 Make a loose fist and stretch out fingers and thumbs. Do this a few times.

Repeat on the other hand.

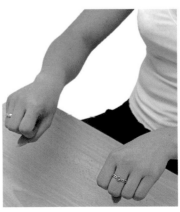

Prayer Stretch

1 Place your palms together in the prayer position. Press palms strongly together, lowering the elbows until they are horizontal.

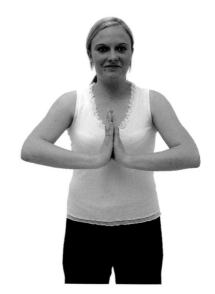

2 Keep lowering your hands until just your fingers press strongly against each other. You should feel a stretch on the inside of the lower arm and wrist. Hold for a breath and return to the starting position.

Repeat two or three times.

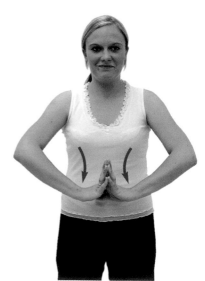

The Flower

You can have fun with this pose and work on your energy centres at the same time, by visualising different-coloured flowers (see page 84).

1 Sit with your spine straight, and the back of your neck long.

2 Holding your hands out in front of you, make them into fists with folded fingers turned to the ceiling, as shown. These are the flowerbuds.

3 Slowly open the fingers like petals, but make your fingers resist against opening up.

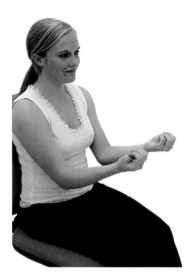

4 Stretch open your fingers and thumbs wide, as shown. Fingers arch slightly backwards.

5 Soften your fingers and turn palms-down. Shake your hands vigorously, as though you are shaking drops of water from the petals.

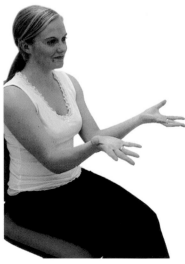

legs & feet

Now that you have worked on the top half of your body, give a little thought to the lower half – legs and feet. With the increased coverage given to air travel and DVT (deep vein thrombosis), it is worth while spending some time focusing on what you can do to keep the circulation flowing in your legs.

Look Good or Feel Good?

How many of us have slavishly followed footwear fashion and squashed our feet into something that looks as though it was never designed to hold a foot, such as spiky high heels or pointy toes? One of the easiest ways of improving your foot health is by wearing comfortable, low-heeled shoes. They mean that you can walk to your heart's content and that you won't be throwing your posture out of alignment.

FEET & LEGS: DO

- get up every hour or so and walk about to stretch your legs.
- sit with legs and knees hip-distance apart, knees at right angles to your shins and feet flat on the floor. If your feet are dangling, adjust your chair or use a foot rest or a couple of phone books.

FEET & LEGS: DON'T

- sit with your legs crossed under your desk as this will constrict the circulation.
- wear high heels that throw your weight forward, jeopardising your posture.
- allow your feet to dangle unsupported in mid air – support them with some kind of foot rest.

Leg Stretch

1 Sit on the edge of your chair, feet flat on floor about one foot apart, feet parallel. Lift out of sitting bones.

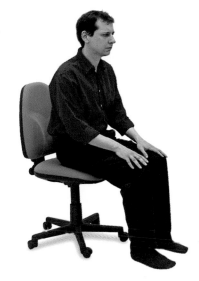

2 Stretch your left leg out in front of you, so that you straighten out leg. Stretch for a total of ten times.

Repeat with your right leg.

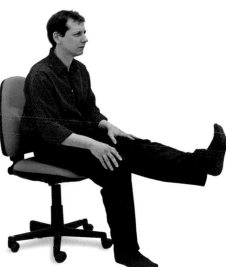

Feet Stretch

1 Sit on the edge of your chair, feet flat on floor about one foot apart and parallel.

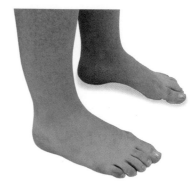

2 Press down on the balls of your feet, lifting heel into air.

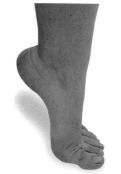

3 Press down on the back of your heels, lifting toes into air.

Repeat eight times.

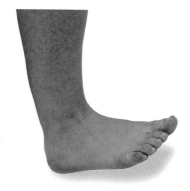

Ankle Circles

1 Sit on your chair, right foot flat on the ground.

2 Lift your left foot across your right thigh.

3 Rotate your ankle clockwise twenty times.

4 Rotate anti-clockwise twenty times.

Repeat the exercise with your right ankle across your left thigh.

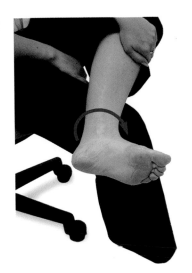

Knee to Chest

1 Sit on the edge of your chair, feet flat on floor about one foot apart, feet parallel.

2 Bend your left knee up towards your chest and place your hands round the leg just below the knee.

3 Pull your knee gently towards your chest, as shown. Hold for a couple of breaths.

Repeat with right knee, holding for a couple of breaths.

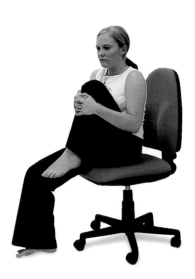

eyes, nose, ears & face

Exercising the Eyes

How many people know that their eyes can be exercised? If your eyes were people, what do you think yours would be like? A finely toned dancer or a couch potato? Many problems with eyesight are caused by eye muscles that have not been kept flexible and healthy. This means that your eyes find it hard to focus at different distances, especially if you spend hours each day working at a computer screen.

Do you ever find that your eyes have become locked into a stare? You are so engrossed in the screen in front of you that you forget to blink. And when you are interrupted or distracted by someone across the room, your vision is fuzzy when you look up?

You need to look after your eyes! Not only exercising them, but relaxing them from the onslaught of activity all around. Have you ever watched a cookery programme filmed with a hand-held camera? The picture is jumping around and you are trying to see what the chef is doing. In the end you have to turn your head away because you find it too unsettling to watch. Your eyes are exhausted just trying to keep up. According to yoga, relaxation is perhaps the most important

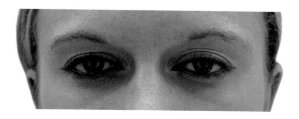

PROBLEMS ASSOCIATED WITH TIRED EYES

- **stinging, dry eyes** from concentrating so hard on the screen that we often forget to blink, causing the eyes to become very dry.
- **tired eyes** caused by spending too long at the computer. Taking screen breaks every half hour or so is a simple solution. Another cause can be bright office lights which contrast with a dimmer computer screen.
- **tension in the eyes** because you are under stress to complete something on screen. You fall into a stare.

element of eye care. By relaxing the eyes you can quieten the mind and improve concentration.

The correct eye level for working on a screen

You should also make sure that your eyes are at the correct level with the computer screen. Otherwise you may be causing neck and shoulder problems. If you are looking up at the screen, then the back of your neck will be scrunched up. If you are looking down at the screen, then the back of your neck is over-stretched with the weight of your head.

The best position is for the top of your screen to be level with your eyes. Your chin will be tucked in and the back of your neck will be long and relaxed. This is the most natural position for the head. It rests gently at the top of the spine not causing any tension in the muscles of the neck and shoulder.

Give Your Eyes a Workout!

There are a number of exercises you can do to keep your eyes in good condition.

Sit in a comfortable position. The back of your neck should be long with your chin tucked in slightly.

Palming

Ideally this is done in darkness so that the eyes can recover from the stress of light.

1 .Rub the palms of your hands lightly together until you feel heat between them.

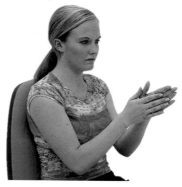

2 Very lightly cup your hands (fingers crossed loosely at your forehead) over your eyes and relax for a few moments.

Visualize this blackness, let it soothe your mind and relax your brain. Breathe deeply and smoothly. Practise for as long is comfortable for you.

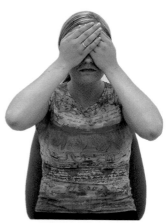

Up & Down Eye Movements

Without moving your head look up to the ceiling, then look down to the floor. Keep your eyes soft and try not to blink.

Repeat ten times and follow with Palming (page 58).

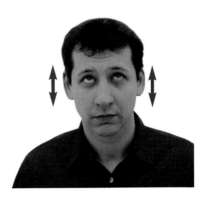

Side-to-Side Eye Movements

Without moving your head, look as far to the right as you can. Then look as far to the left as you can.

Repeat ten times and follow with Palming (page 58).

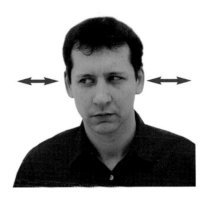

Circular Eye Movements

Roll your eyes round in as big a circle as possible. Do it ten times clockwise, followed by ten times anti-clockwise.

Follow with Palming (page 58).

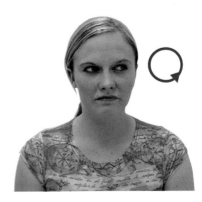

Diagonal Eye Movements

Without moving your head, look up to the top right-hand corner of your right eye and then down to the bottom left-hand corner of your left eye. Repeat ten times.

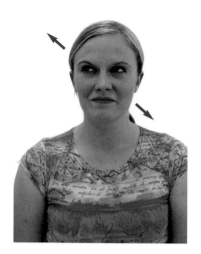

Do the opposite: look up to to top left-hand corner of your left eye and down to the bottom right-hand corner of the right eye. Repeat ten times.

Follow with Palming (page 58).

Blinking

When you are concentrating on work, whether on screen or on paper, you tend to fall into a stare, as though you can't tear your eyes away from what you are doing. This is a strain for the eyes which you can relieve with blinking.

Gently and softly blink the eyes.

This gets rid of any tension in the eyes and keeps them moist.

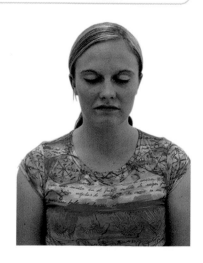

Exercising Your Focus

Far and near, near and far:
Pick a point in the distance to focus on. Straighten your left arm in front of you and stick your thumb up. The tip of the thumb should be just below the point you have been focusing on in the distance.

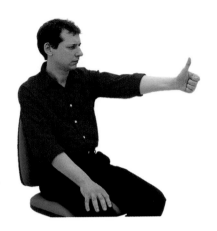

Begin to switch your focus. First look at the faraway point, then look at the tip of your thumb.

Repeat ten times and follow with Palming (page 58).

Coming closer and moving out:
Raise your left arm and stick your thumb up. Take your focus onto the tip of your thumb and keep it there as you bring your thumb slowly to the tip of your nose. Pause for a moment.

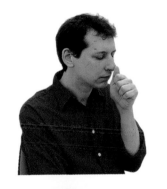

Keep your eye focused on your thumb as you stretch your arm out.

Repeat ten times with a pause in between.

Follow with Palming (page 58).

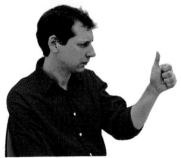

Eye Massage

According to Chinese yoga, the eyes are the opening to your liver and if you suffer from eye problems then you are quite likely to suffer from disorders of the liver. That's the bad news. But the good news is that by practising the following eye exercises you can keep both eyes and liver healthy!

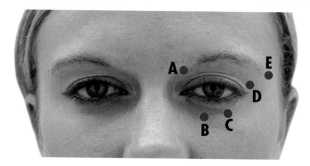

1 Press point A on each eye with the thumbs. You should press quite heavily for about ten seconds. Then rub, again quite heavily, with the thumbs.

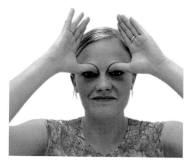

2 Press point B on each eye with the index fingers. You should press quite heavily for about ten seconds. Then rub heavily with the thumbs.

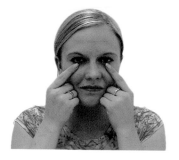

3 Press point C on each eye with the index fingers. You should press quite heavily for about ten seconds. Then rub heavily with the thumbs.

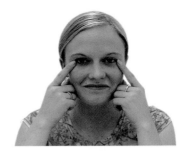

4 Press point D on each eye with the thumbs. You should press quite heavily for about ten seconds. Then rub heavily with the thumbs.

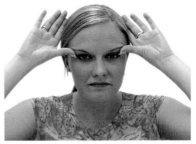

5 Press point E on each eye with the index fingers. You should press quite heavily for about ten seconds. Then rub heavily with the thumbs.

Repeat the whole sequence another two times.

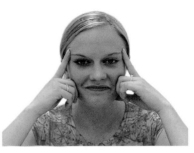

When you have completed this, using your fingers and starting from inside the eyes at the top of the nose, trace the eye socket so that you can feel the bone. Do this for ten seconds. Only go in this direction as going the opposite way causes weakness and wrinkles. Follow with Palming (page 58).

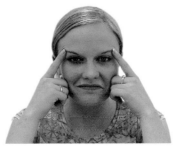

Repeat the whole sequence as often as you like.

Eye Cleansing

In yoga this is traditionally done with a candle. However, you can use any object. You could use a plant or flower or object on your desk. This simple exercise not only cleanses your eyes, it also improves your concentration and clears your mind.

Concentrate your gaze on the object without blinking until your eyes begin to water. Then close your eyes and keep the image of the object in your mind's eye for as long as you can.

As you practise, try to lengthen the time you are able to visualize the object with your eyes shut.

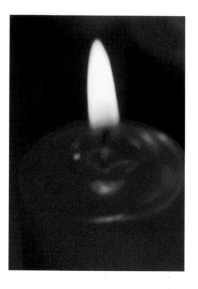

Give Your Ears a Workout!

You may never have thought of exercising your ears! According to Chinese yoga, your ears are the opening to the kidneys. Any problems with your ears may be a sign that there is weakness in your kidneys.

- Placing your index fingers behind each ear flap, fold them over so that you close your ear opening off to the outside. Using the tips of your second fingers, tap on the nails of your index fingers. (You may find this a bit fiddly at first.)

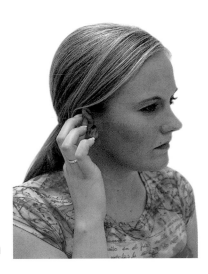

The tapping should sound like the beating of a drum. Do it between 12 and 36 times. Pause and repeat for a further two rounds.

This exercise keeps your ears healthy and can help with problems such as tinnitus.

- Pull your ears upwards as though you wanted to lift your body up by your ears. In the same way, pull the ear lobes downwards. Repeat three times.

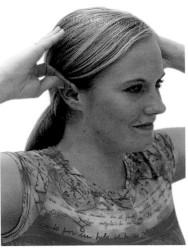

Give Your Nose a Workout!

> According to Chinese yoga, the nose is the opening to the lungs. Allergies, runny noses and blocked sinuses are all thought to be weaknesses in the lungs. We can keep both lungs and sinuses healthy by stimulating certain points around the nose which ensure that the energy flows freely.

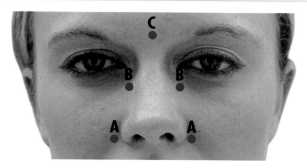

1 Using the tips of your index fingers, press down at point A (just on the outside of the base of each nostril). Press firmly for ten seconds. Then rub these two points with your fingers.

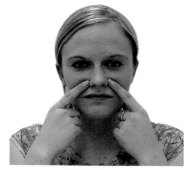

2 Using the tips of your index fingers, press point B firmly for about ten seconds. Then rub these two points with your fingers.

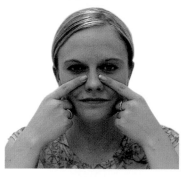

3 Using the tips of your index fingers (one on top of the other) press point C (between your eyebrows) for ten seconds.

Repeat the above sequence another two times starting from point A.

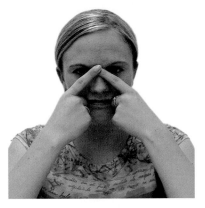

4 Rub through the three points with your index fingers in one continual flow. Repeat another two times, making sure that you press firmly.

These exercises can be practised after the eye exercises on page 59.

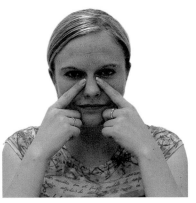

Exercising the Face & Head

Face Exercise

This one is for tired faces! It will also keep wrinkles at bay.

1 As with the Palming routine on page 58, rub the palms of your hands together lightly until you feel heat and energy build up.

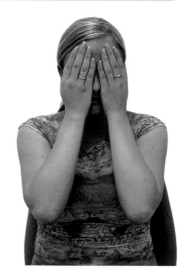

2 Press the palms against your face and visualize this energy being absorbed into your skin.

3 Start rubbing your hands in outward circular movements, bringing hands and fingers up through the bridge of your nose, between your eyebrows and then across the forehead, down your temples and cheeks, across your chin and mouth.

Do it as long as you like and rub your palms together when you feel the warmth going from your hands.

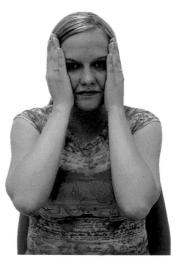

Hair Pulling

> *This one is recommended for hangovers and indigestion!*

Vigorously pull the hair by fistfuls all over the scalp.

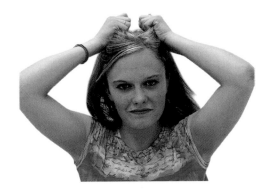

Head Rubbing

Place fingers on the scalp as shown and rub scalp back and forth to stimulate scalp circulation.

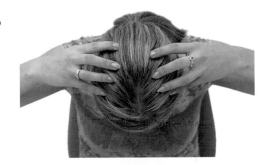

Press the fingers firmly on back of neck as shown and rub the two points. If you are prone to tension headaches, this is an ideal way of ridding any tension in the back of the neck.

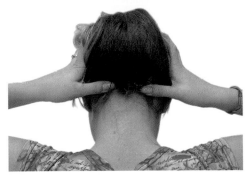

The Lion

If you work in an open-plan office, you may want to choose a private spot for this exercise – or run the risk of giving your colleagues a laugh! This is a good pose to bring blood to the back of the throat and ward off a sore throat. It also stretches the face muscles and muscles around your eyes.

1 Sit on the edge of your chair, feet flat on the ground and hip distance apart. Your spine should be straight and the back of your neck long and relaxed.

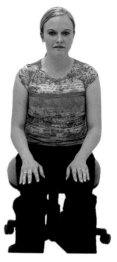

2 Place the palms of your hands on your knees, as shown, with fingers relaxed. Breathe in.

3 Breathing out through the mouth with a quiet roar, come forward, sliding your hands down and stretching out your fingers. At the same time the top of your body moves forward, your mouth opens and you stick your tongue out as far as you can.

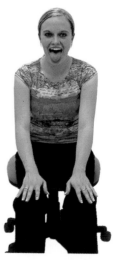

4 As your tongue comes out, open your eyes as wide as they can go. Pause for a moment at the end of the out breath.

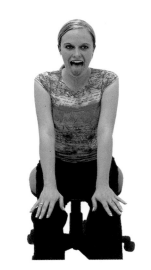

5 Breathing in, return to the starting position.

Repeat a couple of times.

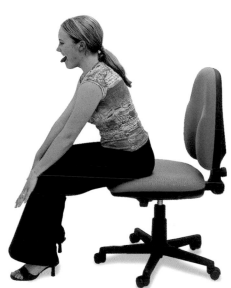

The Lion –
the pose from the side

breathing

Do you ever find that you are so desperate to meet a deadline and concentrating so hard that you have practically stopped breathing? When you finally do finish or take a break, you realize that there has been virtually no movement in your lungs and you need to gulp in some air.

It's strange how this happens, as though you are so fearful of not getting the work done that you hold your breath. Like good posture, breathing is something we seem to unlearn as we grow up. Little by little, we retreat into the upper reaches of the lungs. It's like living your life in the attic, when you have large grand rooms downstairs that you never bother to visit.

As with the spine, it's worth taking a moment to understand how the lungs work and find out what type of breather you are. Then you can begin to put right any bad habits.

How You Breathe

Just as the pelvis plays a major role in your posture, your diaphragm plays a big part in how you breathe.

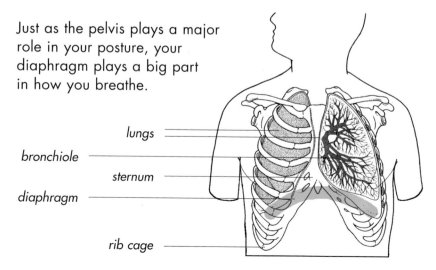

lungs

bronchiole

sternum

diaphragm

rib cage

BENEFITS OF BREATHING CORRECTLY

- *Supplies more oxygen to the body which is vital for it to function.*
- *Removes carbon dioxide, the waste product of any activity.*
- *Removes tension and relaxes the body.*
- *Calms and quietens the mind.*
- *Improves concentration.*
- *Refreshes both the body and mind.*
- *Improves circulation of the blood.*
- *Makes you flourish and look healthy – poor breathers (and smokers) often look drawn and have poor skin tone.*
- *Strengthens the immune system, promoting better health.*
- *Increases the capacity of the lungs.*

The diaphragm is the large, dome-shaped muscle (shown in pink in the illustration opposite) that practically divides the body in two. Above it lie the heart and lungs, below it lie all the other major organs: liver, stomach, kidneys, etc.

When you breathe in, the lungs fill like two balloons, filling up the space in the chest by pushing the ribs outwards and upwards. The diaphragm is pushed down by these expanding lungs. When you breathe out, the lungs deflate like empty balloons, the ribs return back into place and the diaphragm comes back to its original position.

To breathe correctly, you must keep in mind the role of the diaphragm. In order to get it moving, you must ensure that you fill the lowest parts of the lungs, which then push the diaphragm downwards. Just filling the middle portion of your lungs so that your chest sticks out doesn't get your diaphragm moving. It only makes it look as though something is happening.

What kind of breather are you?

Here are some simple tests for you to find out how you breathe – you probably didn't know there could be so many different ways and types! As you have to lie down to do them, they are best done in the privacy of your own home.

Upper-chest breathing Lie on your back. Place one palm lightly on your upper chest and the other on your tummy. Breathe in and out and check what is happening to your hands. If the one on your chest moves, but the one on your tummy stays still, then you are a chest breather. Note how much movement there was in you hand. If it there was hardly any, it is a sign of inefficient breathing. You need to get much more air into all parts of your lungs.

Shallow breathing Lie on your back. Place your hands on each side of your trunk so that you can feel your lower ribs. When you breathe in you should feel your ribs moving out. As you breathe out you should feel them returning to their original position. If you feel no movement, then your breathing is too shallow.

Overbreathing Make sure that you are relaxed and your breathing is natural and at its normal rhythm. Count the length of your next out-breath and compare it to the length of your next in-breath. The out-breath should be slightly longer. If it isn't, then you are an overbreather.

A second test is to shorten your in-breath. If it causes distress, then you are an overbreather. You are in effect hyperventilating and not allowing a chance for carbon dioxide to be removed from your lungs.

Breath-holding To find out whether you hold your breath after breathing in, you have to focus on that point between the end of the in-breath and the beginning of the out-breath. The breath-holder experiences a slight "catch" and has difficulty actually starting the out-breath, as though you don't want to let go of the air in your lungs. This is one of the most common breathing problems.

Reverse breathing This is when the diaphragm goes the wrong way. On the in-breath it is pulled upward and on the out-breath it is pushed down. Lie on your back and place your hands on your tummy. As you breathe out, the tummy should slowly flatten. As you breathe in it should rise gently. If you are doing it the other way around, you are a reverse breather. Try to check whether you are doing it during exercise.

Mouth breathing Do you breathe in and out through the mouth and not the nose? If you do, you are a mouth breather.

BENEFITS OF BREATHING EXERCISES

- *empty lungs fully, getting rid of stale air*
- *lower carbon monoxide*
- *benefit those with asthma or bronchitis*
- *counteract anxiety*
- *purify the nerves*
- *promote good sleep*
- *relax nervous system*
- *aid digestion and liver*
- *purify the nerves*

AVOID BREATHING EXERCISES IF

- *you have abnormal blood pressure*
- *you have heart trouble*
- *the air is very hot or cold*

Changing Your Breathing Habits

You should practise complete breathing. This will give you the blueprint for correct breathing. Once you are aware of bad breathing, as with bad posture, you will always have that little voice nagging at you to put it right.

In order for you to be able to breathe fully, first you need to feel the air filling all the areas of the lungs. We will begin by directing the breath into the three areas of the lungs: lower, middle and upper. Once you can do this, you will find the Complete Breath much simpler to do.

Practise Breathing

1 Place your palms horizontally just above your navel. Fingertips should be touching. Breathing in deeply, direct your breath into your hands. You should feel your fingertips moving away from each other as your diaphragm moves down and gently pushes your belly out.

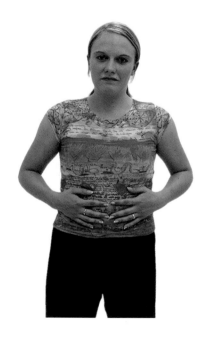

On the out-breath, your fingertips come back together as the diaphragm returns to its normal position and lets your abdomen return to its place. Keep breathing like this until you get a feel for lower or abdominal breathing.

2 Place the palms of your hands at the sides of your body, just below your bust so that you can feel your ribcage (fingers point into your centre). Breathing in deeply, direct your breath into your hands. You should feel your hands being pushed outward.

On the out-breath, your hands return to their starting position. Keep breathing like this until you get a feel for mid-chest breathing.

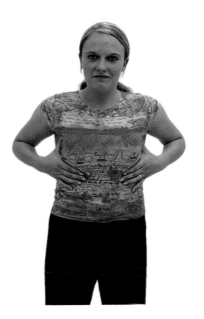

3 Rest the palms of your hands over the tops of your shoulders, fingers facing backward. Breathing in deeply, direct your breath into your hands and see if you can feel them rising and falling slightly as your lungs expand into the space over the backs of your shoulder.

Keep breathing like this until you get a feel for upper chest breathing.

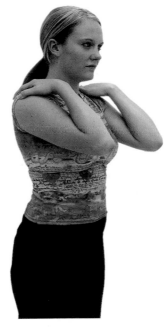

Complete or Full Breathing

This can be practised standing, sitting or lying down. If you do practise it in a sitting position, ensure that your spine is straight with your shoulders back, relaxed and down (see page 15 for correct sitting posture).

1 Begin by emptying the lungs and softly pulling in the tummy muscles to squeeze out any last traces of air from the bottom of the lungs.

2 Relax the tummy muscles and begin breathing in slowly and deeply. Feel the air filling in the lowest parts of the lungs.

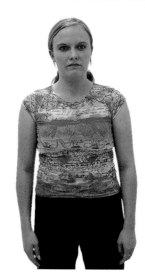

3 Then fill the middle portion of the lungs so that you feel your ribs expanding out to the sides. You can place your hands either side of your ribcage and feel them moving with your ribs.

4 Finally, fill the upper portion of the lungs, beneath the collarbones and over the tops of your shoulders.

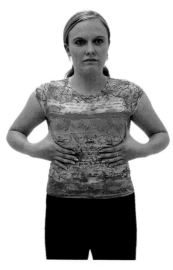

Those expanding lungs can reach parts you never knew existed! Once you are more familiar with the sequence flow from one step to another. Keep your breathing slow and rhythmic. The out-breath should be slightly longer than the in-breath.

5 Pause for a moment at the end of your in-breath, then slowly release the air out of your lungs. Try to do it in the reverse order: first emptying the top of the lungs, then the middle, then the lower lungs, pulling in tummy muscles slightly to squeeze out the bottom traces of air.

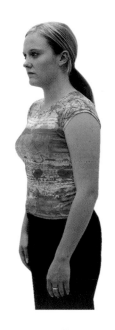

TIP *Visualize a glass jug. When you pour water in, first the bottom fills, then the middle, then the top. When you empty the jug, the water comes out of the top, then the middle, then the bottom. See your lungs as the jug and the water as air.*

Cleansing or Woodchopper Breath

Done either seated and standing, this is good for releasing anger.

1 Stand with feet hip-width apart. Interlock your fingers and raise straight arms above your head.

2 Breathe out through the mouth with a "ha" sound as you bend forward. Arms swing through the legs, as though you were chopping wood. Bend your knees slightly at the same time and pull in abdominal muscles to squeeze out all the air from the bottom of the lungs.

3 Breathe in deeply through the nostrils as you straighten up. Arms come back up over your head. Knees should be slightly bent to protect the lower back.

Repeat three times. As you do so, feel the stale air leaving your lungs and being replaced with clean air.

 Avoid if you have high blood pressure.

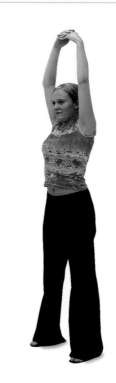

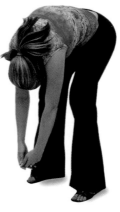

Alternate-Nostril Breathing

1 Sit comfortably with spine straight.

2 Take your right hand and fold the index and middle finger into your palm. (The thumb, fourth and little fingers are straight.)

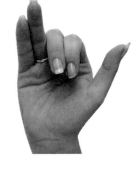

3 Close the right nostril with the thumb and breathe in fully and slowly through the left nostril.

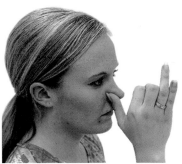

4 Close the left nostril with the fourth and little fingers and breathe out through the right. Pause and then breathe in through the same nostril.

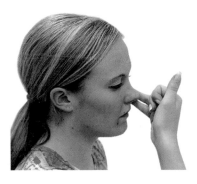

5 Close the right nostril and breathe out through the left.

This completes one cycle and you begin again, inhaling through the left nostril.

Only do three cycles to begin with.

Cooling Breath

1 Begin by breathing regularly.

2 Stick out your tongue and curl it into a tube.

3 Breathe in slowly through the curled up tongue. You will feel the cold air on your tongue.

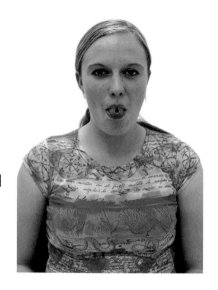

4 Pull your tongue back in and close your mouth.

5 Breathe out slowly through the nose.

Repeat as often as you like.

Note: not everyone can roll their tongue – it's genetic.

How different situations affect breathing

When you are aware how important breathing is for your general good health, you will find yourself paying more attention to it in different situations. Knowing how to breathe properly and what effect your breathing can have will help you both to keep in control during challenging situations and to enhance pleasant ones. Look at the following different emotional and physical states.

BREATHING PATTERNS IN DIFFERENT STATES & EMOTIONS

- **panic or fear** *makes your breathing very fast and shallow, almost a gasping for breath. The rhythm can be erratic.*
- **anger** *makes you take short, sharp breaths.*
- **vigorous exercise** *you take fast, deep breaths to replenish your body with oxygen to fuel the muscles.*
- **contentment** *results in smooth, slow breathing.*

The next time you find yourself in of these states, stop for a moment and take note of how it is affecting your breathing. Then you can take steps to remedy or enhance the situation.

There are a number of other breathing techniques practised in yoga. However, it is better to learn them under the guidance of a trained teacher. If you experience any distress with the breathing exercises you should stop and seek advice from a teacher before carrying on. You can find a teacher from the websites listed on page 93.

unblocking your energy

Do you ever find yourself tired, sluggish and feeling low? You feel like you need a tonic – and not the kind you have with gin! Again, yoga can help.

It is believed that your body contains not only blood, bones and muscles, but also a substance known as *prana*, or subtle energy. This energy is carried through the body via a network of channels. One of the main ones runs along the spine. This is why it is so important to keep your spine healthy and flexible. Breathing also helps to ensure the steady flow of energy around your body.

Along the length of the spine lie energy centres, or wheels (known as *chakras*), to help the energy move upwards and disperse it through your entire body. There are seven energy centres, each with an associated colour. Each is also believed to influence certain aspects of your physical and emotional health. Like a blocked pipe, which can wreak havoc in your home, a block in your energy channel can cause problems.

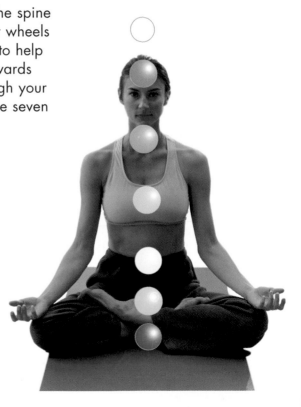

location: crown
colour: white/violet
influences: pineal gland
represents: enlightenment, bliss
imbalance may lead to: psychological problems

location: mid-forehead (3rd eye)
colour: indigo
influences: pituitary gland, nervous system
represents: intuition, wisdom
imbalance may lead to: sinus or eye problems

location: throat
colour: light blue
influences: thyroid, throat, lungs
represents: higher knowledge, learning
imbalance may lead to: sore throat, problems communicating

location: centre of chest (heart)
colour: green
influences: heart, blood circulation
represents: love, compassion, emotions
imbalance may lead to: immune & heart problems, lack of compassion

location: navel (solar plexus)
colour: yellow
influences: digestive system
represents: will power, self-assertion
imbalance may lead to: anger or a sense of victimisation

location: genital area
colour: orange
influences: reproduction, growth
represents: growth, preservation
imbalance may lead to: emotional or sexual problems

location: base of spine (anus)
colour: red
influences: elimination processes
represents: physical strength, stability
imbalance may lead to: paranoia, greed, attachment to things

Balancing Your Energy Centres

- You can do this by focusing your attention on each of the energy centres in turn. As you concentrate on each one, visualize the colour of the centre glowing brightly.

- If you feel out-of-sorts and you can work out which of the energy centres might be in need of a little recharging, focus on that one. You can also help to recharge it by wearing the colour associated with it. It doesn't need to be that full-length violet bridesmaid dress you had hanging in the wardrobe! It could be a scarf or top, or even knickers!

- Move the part of spine affected. Move your pelvis if it is the lower centres that are sluggish. Breathe into the lowest part of your lungs if it is the middle (yellow) energy centre. Do the neck and shoulder exercises for the upper back centres. And for the crown of the head, try visualising a shower of golden light falling over your head and shoulders.

Afterwards, rub the palms of your hands together so that you feel warmth and energy and place them over your eyes (as in the Palming exercise on page 58). This will close down the energy centres and not leave them susceptible to any negative energy. Did you realize there was so much going on around you?

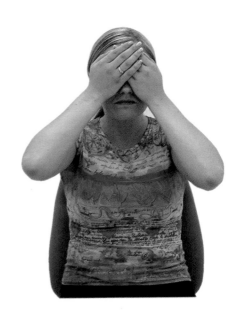

Is Your Desk Clutter Sapping Your Energy?

Energy isn't just within our bodies, it also flows around us. According to feng shui, you need to let this energy flow freely or else it gets caught up and you get bogged down. And everyone knows that a good clear-out does wonders for lifting your spirits and making you feel lighter and more able to get on with tasks.

Unfortunately, modern technology means that we can create even more hidden clutter. Check if your computer needs a good clear-out. Is your e-mail full of messages you could trash or else file away? Try to get into the habit of doing it immediately. Otherwise you create more electronic clutter and probably, like me, spend time wasted scrolling through hundreds of messages trying to find some important information that you ignored when it arrived.

TIPS FOR AN ENERGY-FILLED ENVIRONMENT

- *Clear the clutter from your desk: find a home for everything, so that you can find things in an instant.*
- *Deal with items as they arise: try to get into the habit of not touching a piece of paper twice. This avoids having the task hanging over you, and even forgetting to do it at all.*
- *Keep your computer disks under control: Catalogue and store your disks to avoid wasting time on endless searches for files you need.*
- *Look after your plants: There is nothing so sapping as a wilting plant, seemingly sitting there accusingly and constantly reminding that you aren't looking after it.*
- *Wear loose, comfortable clothing and shoes: Tight waistbands and sore feet drain you of energy.*

TIPS FOR ENERGY-BOOSTING EATING

- *Eat three regular meals a day: heavy-set body types whose digestion is slow, should just have a very light breakfast.*
- *Don't overeat: you should leave a quarter of your stomach empty. The difficult part is recognising when you have reached that point.*
- *Don't eat anything in between meals: if you do need something, make it healthy, like fruit or nuts.*
- *Try not to drink too much tea and coffee.*
- *Drink plenty of water: unless you are the heavy-set body type who needs no extra lubrication and who has probably always struggled with the advice of drinking 2 litres per day.*
- *Eat fresh, natural foods (the ones with most prana or energy): anything that has been overcooked or been around on your shelf for too long, will have little energy left. Hence it is best to eat food that is in season.*
- *Go organic whenever possible, particularly with meat.*
- *Try not to eat too much sugar and refined foods.*
- *Be moderate with your alcohol consumption.*
- *Chew foods thoroughly to extract the goodness and aid digestion.*
- *Try not to have any distractions while you eat: don't eat at your desk, or watch the TV or read. Concentrate on your food – you need to be relaxed and aware of the food going into your mouth. Think of it as munching meditation!*
- *Don't eat foods that are too rich.*

Is Your Diet Sapping Your Energy?

Yoga is about living a balanced healthy life. This applies to what you eat. To know what you should be eating, you have to know your body type and make sure that you eat foods that are in tune with it and not ones that aggravate it. Unfortunately, what you crave for when you are at a low point, is probably the one that is worst for you! To find out what body type you are according to yoga principles, visit the websites on page 93 or see books for further reading on page 95.

Whatever types of food are best for you, the tips on the page opposite can apply to anyone. However, having them is one thing – the challenge is following them. But if you persevere, and are at least aware of what you should be doing, you will always have that little voice nagging at your conscience, setting you back on the yoga path when you stray.

Finally...

The good thing about yoga is that it is not just for 9 to 5 – it's for life! I have just touched on all it has to offer in this book and you will find a wealth of more detailed information in the further reading list on page 95. Although I try to explain the different exercises as fully as possible, nothing beats attending a class. The useful websites on page 93 should be able to point you in the direction of one.

using this book throughout your day

Suggested Routines

The following routines will help you deal with specific conditions or circumstances and help you get the most from this book throughout your day:

Before you start work
• Keyboard warm-ups (page 47)

After a long stretch sitting down
• Leg stretch (page 53)
• Ankle circles (page 55)

After a long stretch on a keyboard
• Hand & wrist exercises 1 (page 43)
• Hand & wrist exercises 2 (page 44)
• Ball squeeze (page 45)

After close-up work on screen
• Palming (page 58)
• Up & down eye movements (page 59)
• Side to side eye movements (page 59)
• Circular eye movements (page 59)
• Diagonal eye movements (page 60)

After a long spell of concentrated work
• Up & down (page 33)
• Side to side (page 34)
• Ear to shoulder (page 35)

- Head circles (page 36)
- Shoulder circles (page 37)

Hunched at your desk for too long
- Chest expander (pages 22–23)
- The blade (page 24)
- Cowface (pages 26–27)

Stiff shoulders
- Forward arm stretch (page 18)
- Vertical arm stretch (page 18)
- Sideways stretch (page 19)
- Upper-arm stretch (page 20)
- Upper-arm stretch and twist (page 20)
- The blade (page 24)
- Cowface (pages 26–27)

Dry eyes
- Eye cleansing (page 64)
- Palming (page 58)

Using headphones or headset too long
- Ear exercises (page 65)

Need to be calm and focused
- Complete breathing (pages 78–79)
- Alternate-nostril breathing (page 89)

Calming down after someone or thing has angered you
- Cleansing or woodchopper breath (page 80)

Need to refresh your energy
- Chair twist (page 29)
- Sitting forward bend (page 31)

The morning after the night before...
• Hair pulling (page 69)
• Head rubbing (page 69)

Working in a stuffy environment
• Nose exercise (pages 66–67)

If you have a tired face and are generally weary
• The lion (pages 70–71)
• Face rubbing (page 68)

Colds and sore throats circulating
• The lion (pages 70–71)

If you are tense and nervous
• Head rubbing (page 69)
• Complete breathing (pages 78–79)

If you are anxious and panicky
• Lower back stretch (page 21)
• Sitting forward bend (page 31)
• Alternate nostril breathing (page 81)

further information

Useful Websites

All the listed websites have links which will take you on very interesting yoga journeys. You can find out lots of useful information from these links and by using a search engine such as Google.

www.bwy.org.uk
British School of Yoga. Includes background information and information about classes for both those who want to attend a class and those who want to become yoga teachers.

www.yogascotland.org.uk
Scottish Yoga Teachers' Association. Includes background information and information about classes for both those who want to attend a class and those who want to become yoga teachers.

indigo.ie/~cmouze
Yoga in Ireland. Information on courses, classes and yoga holidays.

www.viniyoga.co.uk
Details on viniyoga, what it is, courses and classes.

www.yogauk.com
A useful site dedicated to the practice of yoga in the UK. This is the place to come to find a yoga teacher, a yoga event and yoga-related shopping. (You can also read YogaUK online magazine and buy yoga books and videos online from amazon.co.uk)

www.yogajournal.com

A very useful site which includes poses, practices and informative articles which you can print out or send to friends.

www.ayurveda.com
www.ayurvedic.org

Try these two websites if you want to find out a bit more about Ayurveda (well-being) and what your body type is according to the Ayurvedic system

www.bksiyengar.com

Iyengar yoga is the type of yoga taught by BKS Iyengar and teachers who have trained with him.

Further Reading & Sources

The Yoga Thing, Nancy Roberts, Hawthorn Books Inc, 1973

Yoga: 28 Day Exercise Plan, Richard Hittleman, Workman Publishing, 1995

Beat Fatigue with Yoga, Fiona Agombar, Thorsons, 2002

Stretch & Relax, Maxine Tobias & Mary Stewart, Dorling Kindersley, 1988

The Yoga Back Book, Stella Weller, Thorsons, 2000

Stretching, Bob Anderson, Sheleter Publications, Inc, 1980

Light on Yoga, BKS Iyengar, Thorsons, 2001

The Complete System of Chinese Self-Healing, Dr Stephen Chang, Thorsons, 1995

Collins Gem Yoga, Patricia Ralston & C Smart, Harper Collins, 1999

Asana Pranayama Mudra Bandha, Swami Satyananda Saraswati, Yoga Publications Trust, 1996

Office Yoga, Julie Friedeberger, Thorsons, 1991

The Handbook of Ayurveda, Dr Shantha Godagama, Kyle Cathie, 2001

index of exercises

4\23